AF798360

The Successful Clinical Manager - Home Health

Companion Workbook

Copyright

ISBN 978-1-955837-13-2

Published 2022 Deep Creek Publishers

Legal Disclaimer

The author and the publisher of this work have made every effort to ensure the accuracy of information contained within at the time of publication and shall have no liability or responsibility to any person, or entity for any losses or damages incurred, or alleged to have been incurred directly or indirectly by the information contained in this book. The author or publisher make no warranties, expressed or implied, with respect to its content and no warranties may be created or extended by sales representatives, or written sales materials. The author or publisher have no responsibility for the consistency or accuracy of URLs and content of third-party websites referenced in this book. The author and publisher recommend that the reader always consult current regulations, applicable research, and institutional policy and procedures.

The publisher and the author make no guarantees concerning the level of success you may experience by following the advice and strategies contained in this book, and you accept the risk that results will differ for each individual. The testimonials and examples provided in this book show exceptional results, which may not apply to the average reader and are not intended to represent or guarantee that you will achieve the same or similar results.

The publisher and the author do not make any guarantee or other promise as to any results that may be obtained from using the content of this book. You should never make any investment decision without first consulting with your own financial advisor and conducting your own research and due diligence. To the maximum extent permitted by law, the publisher and the author disclaim any and all liability in the event any information, commentary, analysis, opinions, advice and/or recommendations contained in this book prove to be inaccurate, incomplete or unreliable, or result in any investment or other losses.

Also by the Author

- The Successful Clinical Manager – Home Health
- The Successful Clinical Manager – Hospice
- The Successful Clinical Manager – Hospice – Companion Workbook

The Clinical Manager Role Today

The role that the clinical manager in Home Health fulfills is essentially the same when comparing the small agency to the larger agency. Often, the smaller the agency, the larger the span of responsibility of the clinical manager, managing everything from intake to quality. The overall role is one of great importance to the agency. It's what happens between the clinical manager and their staff that moves the agency forward. I like to refer to the job as being the linchpin of the agency. The linchpin is the very important piece of sturdy metal that holds the wheels on a vehicle. If the linchpin breaks or is otherwise faulty, the wheel falls off and the entire operation can come off the rails. The analogy holds true in the role of clinical manager. If it's not working right, there are bound to be problems!

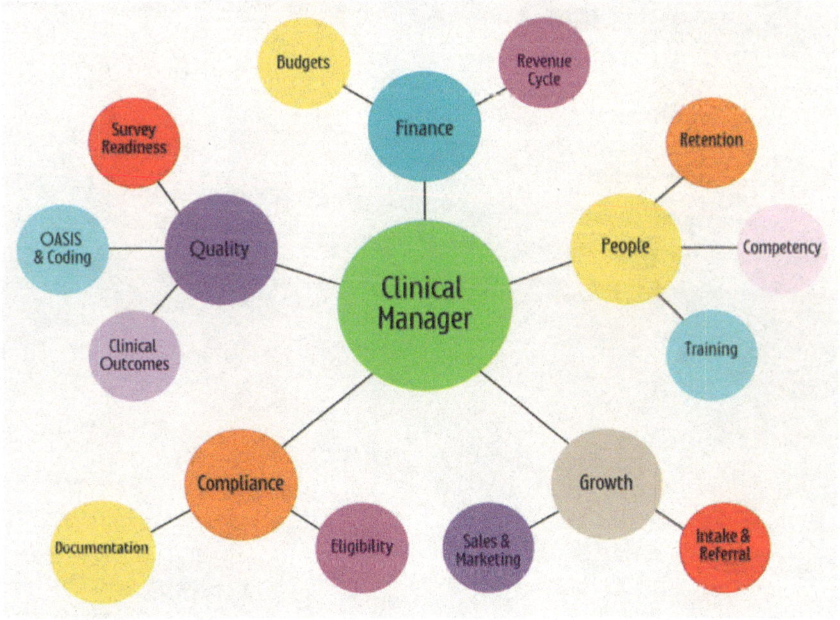

If you are currently in the role of supervisor or clinical manager. List out the job responsibilities that you have.

Knowing Your Own Strengths and Weaknesses

Congratulations on beginning a journey to expand your skill set and knowledge about being a clinical manager! Depending on your experience and time in the role, this journey may be long, or it may be short. But any trek will require those first few steps, and it's here that you need to establish goals to end up where you intended. This is a personal reflection. Maybe you are required to take this course for work, or you are taking it for personal growth reasons or simply you just want to make life a little easier. Whatever the reasons for reading the first lines, let's set out what you want to get out of this journey. These may change as we move through the subject areas, so no worries. There is not one right answer, and your reasons will differ from others.

- Establish long-term goals for yourself. Long term, what is your end game? Where do you want to end up? (This could be anything from learning to read financial statements to becoming the CEO of the agency)

- Set out your short-term goals. What are the immediate steps you need to take to be successful in your role? (We'll be re-looking at this at the end of the book)

- What are some of the qualities you've valued in other managers you've worked with? List them here.

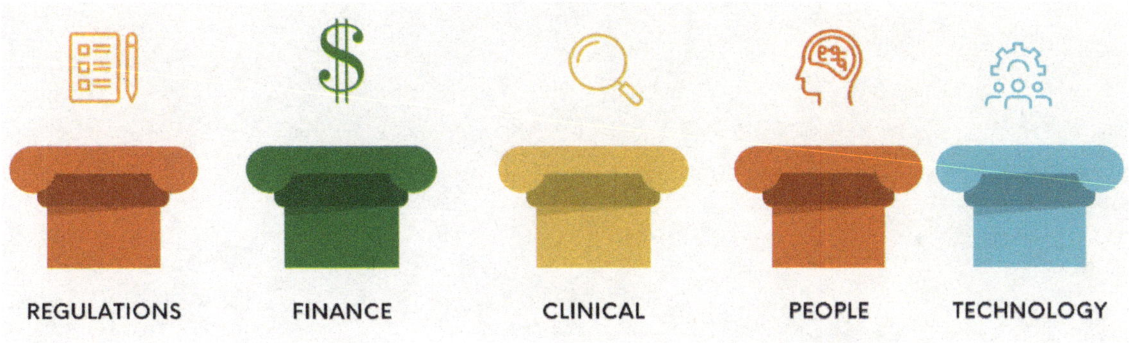

- Looking at the 5 Pillars©–Regulations, Finance, Clinical, People and Technology–where do you feel you need to focus the most?

- Know your weaknesses. Build on a plan to address them and turn them into your strengths. Facing them head on is the best way to get through the challenge. Considering the five pillars, what are the areas you need to focus on? We'll re-visit this when we build your plan. Identify them here.

Regulations Pillar

Overview

There are a ton of regulations to know and follow in home health. There are federal Conditions of Participation (CoPs), state rules and additional regulations for privacy, fraud, OASIS, etc. While you need to have a working knowledge of the regulations, you also need to have resources on hand to look up when needed. All the experts have resources at hand and can reference them frequently. Make sure you have a listing of the rules that apply to you and the links to the most up-to-date resources.

- *Review the tutorial and download the listing of these important links to regulation and resources. Save this to your computer or somewhere you can readily access it and can click a link as needed.*

✓ ☐

Check the box when you've completed the tutorial, downloaded and saved the tool with the important links. (*If you're like me, you can't live with an unchecked box–something important left undone!)*

- *If your state has its own rules for home health, look them up online and collect the link. You do this by copying and pasting the state rules in the search bar onto your desktop as a saved favorite.*

Requirements–Reviewing the Start-Up Process

Starting up a home health agency takes a long time–it can be up to 2 years–although some new agencies have seen a shorter turnaround time. The new entity will see patients without reimbursement for a time–so it's not a process for the faint hearted and requires resources to pay staff and maintain the entity prior to Medicare certification. Some states will have specific requirements, such as a Certificate of Need (CON) where the intended new agency will need to prove that there is a need for new services in the area.

Considering your state, is there a CON process for a home health agency? You will need to do some research on your own to find out. Google can be your friend sometimes!

State with CONs will require the agency to submit data regarding the need for another home health agency. This usually considers demographics, hospitalizations, use of long term care facilities and a review of the current home health providers in the area. This review process is a good idea regardless of whether there is a CON law. Why do you think it would be a good idea to understand the marketplace before opening an agency?

How many home health agencies can you name in your area that you compete with? Aside from competing for patients, is there also a competition for staff?

Does your state have rules for home health agencies? Name a few areas that the rules differ from Medicare rules–if at all.

Is your agency accredited? if not what accreditation body are you familiar with? The choices are the Joint Commission, Accreditation Commission for Health care (ACHC), the Community Health Accreditation Partnership (CHAP). Name a few ways that the accrediting rules differ from Medicare rules.

- *OASIS–Do you know how soon the OASIS data has to be transmitted to the QIES system? What is the timeframe?*

- *Do you know the process for OASIS Transmission in your agency? Who has the responsibility to take care of that in your agency?*

- *HIPAA Rules. What are some processes that are used at your agency to ensure compliance with the HIPAA rules? (Hint: look at the annual training requirements)*

- *HHCAHPS–Do you know who your agency uses as a vendor? Have you reviewed the reports? Have you accessed the Compare Website to check out the agencies in your area? (go ahead and do so).*

- *Do you know where your agency policies & procedures are? Do you have easy access to them when needed? Have you read through them?*

Self-Assessment–

This section of the regulations is pretty full of detail. Don't get discouraged! Take a deep breath and write down areas you feel you want to have further information on, re-review, discuss with other colleagues or experts.

Deep Dive into Regulations

Name the 5 requirements for certification of a patient in home health. What are the requirements? (Answers are in the Appendix)

1. ______________________________
2. ______________________________
3. ______________________________
4. ______________________________
5. ______________________________

Name the criteria for Homebound

Criteria One

____

____

____

____

Criteria Two

____

____

____

____

What are some things that a skilled nurse can do under home health? (Chapter 7 - Section 40.1)

What is it about a patient's condition that would qualify them for skilled therapy services rather than just having a home health aide do exercises with a patient? (Chapter 7 40.2.1)

What makes up Maintenance Therapy? What kind of scenario would we be likely to see for a patient requiring Maintenance Therapy?

Do you understand the processes for obtaining orders at your agency? Review the policy in your organization about MD/Allowed provider orders. Review Section 30.2.3 Chapter 7 Specificity of Orders. Is this order written correctly? What's wrong with it?

> *SN 2 to 3 x a week for assessment of cardiac status, lung sounds, vitals and medication teaching of new prescriptions.*

- You can access resources offered by the Medicare Administrative Contractors (MAC) as a good source of further information. Remember, you don't need to be in that MAC's region to access their services–so depending on the areas you want to review further–one MAC may be better than the other.

The Medicare Administration Agencies (MAC)

-Each MAC is a little different–but they all offer education and resources. You CAN access these resources even though the MAC does not cover your area.

- **Palmetto MAC for HH + H** for the following states: Alabama, Arkansas, Florida, Georgia, Illinois, Indiana, Kentucky, Louisiana, Mississippi, New Mexico, North Carolina, Ohio, Oklahoma, South Carolina, Tennessee, and Texas
  - https://www.palmettogba.com/palmetto/jmhhh.nsf/DID/9C6RZ83761
- Palmetto's Local Coverage Determinations (LCDs) (both Home Health & Hospice)
  - https://www.palmettogba.com/palmetto/jmhhh.nsf/DID/8B3RW86238
- Top Claim Denial Reasons for both Home Health & Hospice
  - https://www.palmettogba.com/palmetto/jmhhh.nsf/DID/B9KPVS3022
- **National Government Services (NGS) HH** + H for the following states: Alaska, American Samoa, Arizona, California, Guam, Hawaii, Idaho, Michigan, Minnesota, Nevada, New Jersey, New York, Northern Mariana Islands, Oregon, Puerto Rico, US Virgin Islands, Wisconsin and Washington, Connecticut, Maine, Massachusetts, New Hampshire, Rhode Island, and Vermont
  - https://www.ngsmedicare.com/web/ngs
- NGS's Local Coverage Determinations (LCDs) (both Home Health and Hospice)
  - https://www.ngsmedicare.com/web/ngs/medical-policies?lob=93618&state=97282&region=93623

- **CGS** HH + H for the following states: Delaware, District of Columbia, Colorado, Iowa, Kansas, Maryland, Missouri, Montana, Nebraska, North Dakota, Pennsylvania, South Dakota, Utah, Virginia, West Virginia, and Wyoming
    - https://www.cgsmedicare.com/hhh/
- CGS Local Coverage Determinations
    - https://www.cgsmedicare.com/hhh/coverage/index.html

Knowledge Growth in Regulations

After going through this section on the regulations, where do you find you need to build your knowledge base? List the areas. Keep in mind your long term goal, as well as your current needs. List them here.

What is your plan to address your learning needs?

Finance Pillar

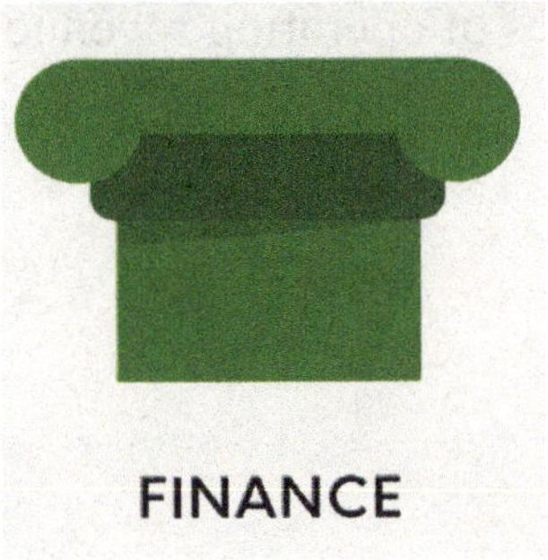

Many folks in clinical management or leadership positions struggle with finance and it raises the stress level of everyone when we talk about money. Largely, the stress comes from feeling inadequate or solid in understanding the ins and outs of finance. I want to help fix that for you, reduce your stress by building a foundation of knowledge you can build on. Understand that your agency, whether it be a for profit privately owned, publicly traded or a non-profit VNA, needs to have money coming in the door in order to function. Whether or not we like it, we are working at a business with taxes to pay and payroll to meet. Our success or failure in managing the money at our agency drives whether we can stay in business. This is like our own personal finances. If we have money coming in, we can afford our mortgage or rent. If we don't, we are sleeping on the couch at a friend's house. The goal for money management, of course, is to have enough left over to focus on growth or new technology. Similar to our personal lives, where we strive to have enough left over for vacations to Disney World or other goals.

To understand the money aspects of a home health agency you need to understand the overall revenue and expense flows.

Revenue

- What are the major sources of operating revenue for your agency?

- Describe some of the non-operational revenue that your agency has, if any. Donations (non-profit), grants, etc.

- Do you know your payer mix? The mix of insurance that the patients on service have, Medicare, Medicaid, Commercial Insurance etc. Be sure to clarify for yourself if any of the payers are managed, need authorizations and pay the agency either per visit or episodically. Describe the payer mix at your agency as far as you are aware.

Revenue Cycle

- Describe what happens from the revenue cycle perspective in each of these steps of the billing cycle
    - **Intake**
    - **Scheduling**
    - **Clinical Care**
    - **Verification** (OASIS, Coding, Authorizations & Plan of Care Review)

- **Pre-Bill**

- **Billing**

Expenses

Staffing and related expenses are the largest portion of expense for a home health or hospice agency. List the areas included when we refer to staffing costs. Remember, it's not just salaries.

Staffing

- Do you know the number of FTEs that you are allocated if you have a team? If you don't, how can you locate that information?

- Make a list of your staff and their FTE. If you have staff that are per diem or casual, make a note of that and see if you can determine their usual FTE worked. This may be hard for some if they only work rarely, but for some of the 'regular' staff, this may be easy to do. Note any open positions. (Suggest that you may want to have this list outside of the workbook as a working document)

- What is your expected productivity by position? How is this calculated at your agency? Are certain visits weighted?

- Why is measuring productivity important?

Turnover

- Do you know the turnover at your agency? Do you know how the agency trends? Do you know how they compare with the average turnover nationally by discipline?

- Why do you think turnover is a concern for expense management?

Key Performance Indicators

- What are the measures you look at monthly or weekly?

- Do you have benchmarks to compare to?

- How does your team compare? If you don't compare favorably in a specific area, do you know why? If not, how are you going to find that information out?

- What does your agency use if anything to benchmark against? If you have nothing or don't know, how will you plan to find out and compare your performance?

The Patient Driven Grouper Model of Payment - PDGM

Much of the revenue in a home health agency is driven by how Medicare pays for care. The Patient Driven Grouper Model (PDGM) has been in effect for a couple of years now and is still considered the new model of payment. As a clinical manager, it is vital that you understand the model and how it works. The provision of care and utilization of visits in an episode is very much on the plate of the clinical manager. High-quality care and clinical outcomes need to be balanced with reimbursement.

The Patient Driven Grouper Model (PDGM) separates payment for a home health episode into two 30-day ***periods***. The ***episode*** for a patient remains at the 60-day mark, with the Plan of Care (POC) or 485 covering the 60-day episode of care.

There are 432 case mix groups for a patient to come under. The groups are determined by the patient's admission source, timing, primary diagnosis and some secondary co-morbidities, and their functional score. It's the completion of the OASIS assessment that drives the overall determination, as well as the admission source. Following is the visual of the PDGM payment model.

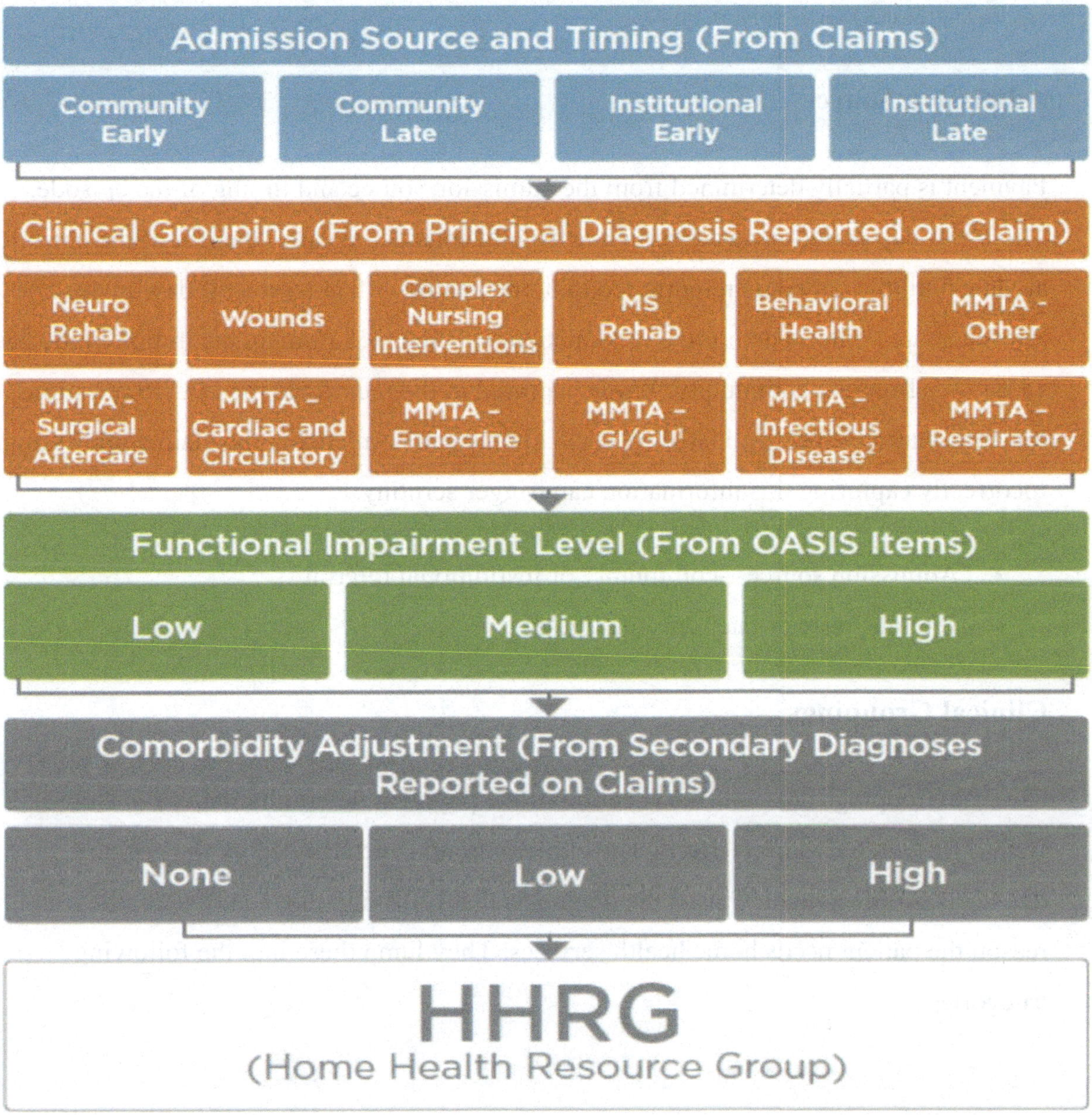

Under the Patient-Driven Groupings Model, a 30-day period is grouped into one (and only one) subcategory under each larger colored category. A 30-day period's combination of subcategories places the 30-day period into one of 432 different payment groups.

1 Gastrointestinal tract/Genitourinary system
2 The infectious disease category also includes diagnoses related to neoplasms and blood-forming diseases

*Source: MLN Matters Number: SE19027, 2019

Admission Source

Payment is partially determined from the admission source and timing of the episode. The 1st 30-day period in an admission is usually considered early, the rest of the episodes are late until the patient is re-admitted to home health with at least a 60-day break. The referral source criteria determine if the patient was referred from an institution in the past 14 days or from the community. While captured in the record via the OASIS questions, this information is also validated by CMS claims and corrected in the claims processing. Incorrectly capturing this information can trigger scrutiny.

- Admission source—community or institutional referral
- Timing–early or later episode timing

Clinical Groupings

Clinical Groupings drive the next section of the payment determination or the Home Health Resource Group (HHRG). The clinical group is determined by the primary diagnosis for the patient. This is the diagnosis that is driving the plan of care, the primary reason the patient needs home health services. They lump these into the following categories.

Clinical Groups	The Primary Reason for the Home Health Encounter is to Provide:
Musculoskeletal Rehabilitation	Therapy (physical, occupational or speech) for a musculoskeletal condition
Neuro/Stroke Rehabilitation	Therapy (physical, occupational or speech) for a neurological condition or stroke
Wounds – Post-Op Wound Aftercare and Skin/Non-Surgical Wound Care	Assessment, treatment & evaluation of a surgical wound(s); assessment, treatment & evaluation of non-surgical wounds, ulcers, burns, and other lesions
Behavioral Health Care	Assessment, treatment & evaluation of psychiatric conditions, including substance use disorder
Complex Nursing Interventions	Assessment, treatment & evaluation of complex medical & surgical conditions including IV, TPN, enteral nutrition, ventilator, and ostomies

Clinical Groups	The Primary Reason for the Home Health Encounter is to Provide:
Medication Management, Teaching and Assessment (MMTA)-- • **MMTA –Surgical Aftercare** • **MMTA – Cardiac/Circulatory** • **MMTA – Endocrine** • **MMTA – GI/GU** • **MMTA – ID/Neoplasms/ Blood Diseases** • **MMTA –Respiratory** • **MMTA – Other**	Assessment, evaluation, teaching, and medication management for a variety of medical and surgical conditions not classified in one of the above listed groups. The subgroups represent common clinical conditions that require home health services for medication management, teaching, and assessment.

*Source: MLN Matters Number: SE19027, 2019

Functional Status

Next is the determination of the functional status. These items are determined through the assessment on the OASIS. Remember that it is the accuracy of the documentation that determines payment. As a clinical manager in home health, it is vital that your staff are doing an accurate ***assessment*** and not an ***interview*** with the OASIS items of function. It's not what the patient says they can do–it's what the clinicians assess that the patient can do! The following are the items in the OASIS that drive the functional score.

OASIS Items from which the Functional Score is derived in PDGM
M1800: Grooming
M1810: Current Ability to Dress Upper Body
M1820: Current ability to Dress Lower Body
M1830: Bathing
M1840: Toilet Transferring
M1850: Transferring
M1860: Ambulation/Locomotion
M1032: Risk of Hospitalization

*Source: MLN Matters Number: SE19027, 2019

Co-Morbidities

Co-morbidities also drive payment for the patient. There are a select bunch of diagnosis that paired with the primary diagnosis will create a higher payment. CMS determined through its research that these diagnoses' groupings would have a higher use of resources in home health and, therefore, would qualify for a higher payment. Patients with these diagnosis combinations would likely need to use more nursing, therapy and aide services.

It's actually really fascinating stuff to read if you have the time. These details are in the Federal Register when the rules are published.

The Co-morbidities are High, Low and None.

- Low = there is a secondary diagnosis that triggers a higher payment
- High = there would be two or more diagnoses on the record that interact and trigger a higher payment
- None = Speaks for itself

Home Health Resource Group

Of interest is that your software systems have to be built around the payments with the correct groupers to calculate these items which determine your overall payment. There is no one in the back office that manually does this, although it is possible to do. Not a job for me! Below is a grid which shows the HHRG number and letter combinations. For example, a 2CC11–would be a patient admitted from a hospital without another home health episode in the 60 days prior, in the wound category, with high functional needs and no comorbidities.

Position #1	Position #2	Position #3	Position #4	Position #5
Source & Timing	Clinical Group	Functional Level	Co-Morbidity	Placeholder
1 - Community Early	**A** - MMTA Other	**A** - Low	**1** - None	**1**
2 - Institutional Early	**B** - Neuro Rehab	**B** - Medium	**2** - Low	
3 - Community Late	**C** - Wounds	**C** - High	**3** - High	
4 - Institutional Late	**D** - Complex Nursing Interv.			
	E - MS Rehab			
	F – Behavioral Health			
	G – MMTA Surgical Aftercare			
	H – MMTA Cardiac & Circulatory			
	I – MMTA Endrocine			
	J – MMTA GI/GU			
	K – MMTA Infectious Disease			
	L – MMTA Respiratory			

*Source: MLN Matters Number: SE19027, 2019

Low Utilization Payment Adjustments

A Low Utilization Payment Adjustment (LUPA) is where the payment for the care provided is on a *per visit* basis instead of an *episodic* basis. This means that instead of being paid by the 30-day period, for example, $2,000, the payment would be $200 for each visit. The payment varies by discipline, nursing, therapy, etc. LUPA thresholds, or limits, range from 2 to 6 visits and are determined by the patient's HHRG. If the threshold for their HHRG is 4, we can provide 4 visits and still be paid for the *full* episode. If we did 3 visits, it would be a considered a LUPA. We don't like LUPAs because the reimbursement rarely covers the cost of care provided. But we take them in the mix of patients.

LUPA management is something a clinical manager should pay close attention to. In PDGM, we are seeing LUPAs becoming a problem on the 2nd period in a 60-day episode. Yes–we have two chances in home health to have a LUPA in the 60-day episode. Sometimes they can be avoided if we manage patients and know when we are in the LUPA range with our care planning. Every visit has to have a skill to be billable, so don't game the system. It will cause claim denials in the long run. Just be aware of practices on your team. Some things you can control are; making sure the case manager is knowledgeable and sees the patient prior to the 30-day mark to determine if they need to go into the 2nd period. Technology should help us by now to see where we are in the episode and make this process easier for the clinicians in the field, however they need to know *why* they are looking at this and the impact to the agency. Training and coaching for the clinicians in PDGM will help in managing successfully in the periods.

Knowledge Growth in Finance

Make a list of the areas you feel you need more help in. Are they revenue? Revenue cycle? Budgeting? Expense management? Deciphering the reports you have for your role?

How are you going to address your learning needs? Meet with the financial person at your organization? Meet with the revenue cycle team?

Areas needing attention:

What would be your plan to address your learning needs?

Clinical Pillar

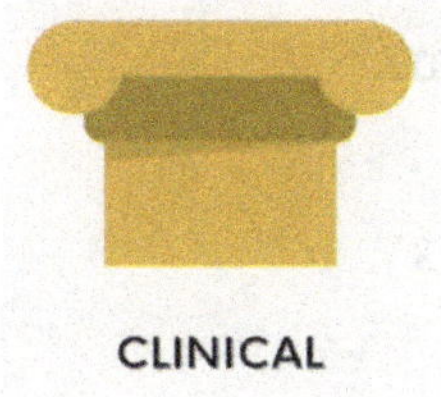

As a clinical manager, most agencies expect that you have come into the role with some level of clinical knowledge in the home health or hospice arena. As a licensed clinician as the federal rules require, you must at least have had enough experience and training to pass the licensure requirements. The federal regulations require:

"§484.115 (c) provides that a clinical manager must be a licensed physician, physical therapist, speech-language pathologist, occupational therapist, audiologist, social worker, or a registered nurse."

As mentioned in the Regulations chapter of this book, states may have more stringent requirements for the role of a clinical manager with further education and experience requirements. Most organizations will require a certain level of experience either from a clinical standpoint or managerial standpoint. Ideally, the minimal requirement should be a substantiative 3-to-5-year experience as a clinician in home health or hospice and at least one year of supervisory experience. Having an acute care background and home health or hospice experience would be ideal, giving a well-rounded clinical experience.

However, in these times in 2022, these key positions are hard to fill. I can honestly say that I have not seen the level of recruitment and advertising out there for clinical managers across the country until recently. It is likely agencies will make concessions to get positions filled, and ambitious folks with little experience will take the role of clinical manager. If that is you, or someone you know, I'm glad you've picked up this book! It's that sink or swim approach to filling open clinical manager positions that prompted the creation of the book and courses at The Clinical Manager Source (http://theclinicalmanagersource.com).

Clinical Policies and Procedures

- It is a best practice to have clinical policies and procedures readily available for the staff and for yourself to use in caring for or directing the staff on the care of patients. Does your agency have clinical policies and procedures? Are they readily accessible for the staff and for yourself? Do you know what's in them and when to resource them? If the answer is no to any of these, specify your plans.

In order to be well prepared and ensure you have the right resources at your fingertips, you need to understand who your agency serves. Identifying what type of clinical needs they have, and determine how you can work to ensure your staff are prepared to provide top-notch care. Knowing the most common conditions, diagnosis, home treatments (wounds, ortho, post stroke etc.) can help you plan specific education or competencies to better serve your patient population. Before jumping in on your own to dig up data about your service area, check within your organization to see if some data mining has already been done.

- What does your patient population look like? Do you have a larger population of patients with certain conditions or diseases?

- How are your staff prepared to care for that patient population? Look at the competencies you are using for orientation and annual evaluations. Are these aligned with the needs of the patient population? If not, what would be your plan to change them?

Knowledge Growth in Clinical Practice

Knowing that the success of your staff will reflect directly back to you as their manager, their success is your success. Where do you need to grow clinically and/or have available for the team and your self as a resource or a training? Where can you bolster the clinical care of your team to better meet the needs of the patients served?

What is needed?

What is the plan to get it?

People Pillar

Managing people effectively is another of the pillars of knowledge that a clinical manager needs to possess. This is likely to be one of the hardest, easiest, most challenging and stimulating of all the pillars. There will be days it seems everyone is troublesome on your team, and days that you wonder if you're suited for management because of the struggles with staff. Really, the job would be so easy if there were no staff and no patients! Then there are the days when everything is clicking, and things are working as they should.

- Evaluate your skillset in knowing how to select and hire people for your team. How comfortable are you in deciding what your team needs for a skillset? How are your interview skills? Do you feel confident interviewing candidates? Do you feel you are skilled in the interview process and can gain adequate information to make a good hiring decision?

- As a manager, you really need to know the personnel policies for your agency. Do you have access to the policies, have read them and have them as a quick reference when needed? Have you established a relationship with the human resource staff covering your team?

Managing People

- Do you know your organization's policy on the disciplinary process of staff? Do you know the steps to take if you have to discipline someone? Are there any special forms you are required to complete in this process?

- What is their process & requirement for the documentation of counseling with employees?

- Coaching an employee can be done as a measure prior to stepping into counseling, but it can also be the fun stuff where you help someone to grow. Ask yourself–how are you with coaching the staff? Note your strengths and weaknesses.

- Do you know the steps to take with terminating an employee? If not, locate this for your organization and review closely. It's important that you are familiar with this process as it can be full of pitfalls. Talk with the HR staff if you have specific questions.

- What are your communications processes with the team? Are they effective?

- What are your communication processes with your superiors? What needs to improve to show your team’s performance?

Managing Yourself

When you became a clinical manager, the role gave you a set of responsibilities and a role to fill. It didn't take away your ability to be human and certainly have feelings and emotions. What it does do is it brings to light the fact that you'd have to have self awareness and control over your emotions.

- How did you score on the emotional intelligence test? Do you need to improve or focus on any aspect? This may take some work to improve your score. What is your plan to address?

- Make notes for yourself on qualities that are strengths and those you'd like to improve.
    - Self Awareness
    - Self Regulation
    - Empathy for others
    - Motivation
    - Social skills

Knowledge and Skill Growth in People Pillar

Managing people and managing yourself are skills you need to continue to grow throughout your career. Make a list of the areas in which you need to grow. Are they in coaching and counseling employees? The hiring processes and interview skills?

What is your plan to address these areas you need more skill with?

Technology Pillar

Technology is the last of the pillars of knowledge for the clinical manager. This pillar has the true underpinning of all the pillars and all the operations in the agency. Technology touches everything we do and has a role in every area of operations. It's important that the clinical manager have a level of comfort and skill with the software in use at the level of a super-user. This skill is valuable in that you are often the front line for staff when they have usage issues and you can influence the correct and best use of the system.

- Evaluate your own skills regarding technology–are you a superuser? Do you feel comfortable with the technology that you use now? If not, what will be your next steps?

- Are you able to function with the system–run your own reports?

- How well can you use the scheduling functions for your team?

- Are you comfortable with the use of the software?

Knowledge Growth in Technology

Do you have areas of weakness when it comes to the overall use if technology and software? Do you work outside your system routinely? List them here.

If you have some areas of weakness, formulate a plan to address these. How can you gain some expertise with the software and grow your level of comfort?

Sales, Intake and Scheduling

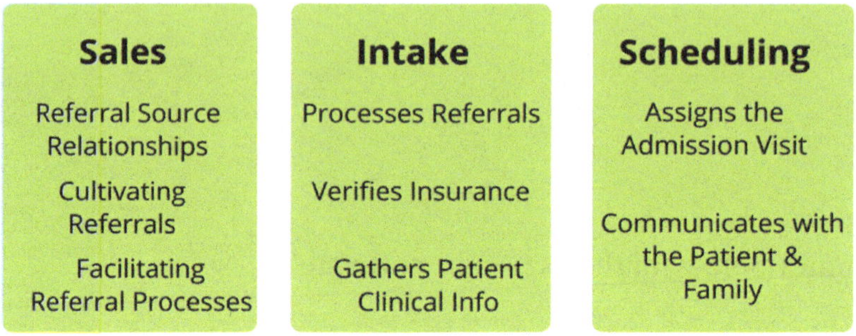

Sales and clinical teams will often have a push pull relationship. The sales team is looking to admit and grow the patient census and the clinical team is trying to meet the needs of all the patients on service. It's important for the clinical manager to understand the role of sales in the agency.

Sales

- Consider your relationship with the sales and liaison team at your organization. What is your relationship? Do you know their growth goals and targets?

- Is there regular communication? If yes, what does that look like?

- Do they need guidance from you on how to manage within the regulations? Are there opportunities for them to better understand your operations?

- Are there opportunities for you to speak with the sales/liaison teams? Maybe a training or a coordination with a specific complex case being referred? A case study?

Intake

The intake process involves the gathering of patient information to move the referral along. Speed and accuracy here are paramount to the prevention of re-work for the clinical team. Data entering demographics and verifying insurance coverage are the main tasks for an intake department. This may sound pretty simple, but there are challenges along the way.

- Considering your current work situation, what is your involvement in the intake department? Do you have a relationship with the leader or someone that handles your team's referrals?

- Do you meet regularly to resolve patient issues, such as lack of information or insurance authorization delays? Work to understand the issues with the insurance companies, verification, and authorization processes.

- How does the initial insurance authorization and the obtaining of re-authorizations work for your agency? (we'll revisit this in the revenue cycle)

Scheduling

Scheduling drives everything in the agency. This is the coordination of people to patients, getting the staff front and center to do the most important part of their job, taking care of patients. Scheduling is also where the clinical manager needs to spend a lot of oversight time to ensure patients are being seen and the staff are being used effectively and efficiently.

- Ensure your oversight of the schedule for your team. Are you looking at it and giving direction to schedulers?

- Ensure a daily plan for taking admissions. Determine if there are trending days for the volumes of admissions. Make accommodations for this.

- Ensure you have an established routine for schedule oversight. Get comfortable with the scheduling processes in the software.

The Care Team

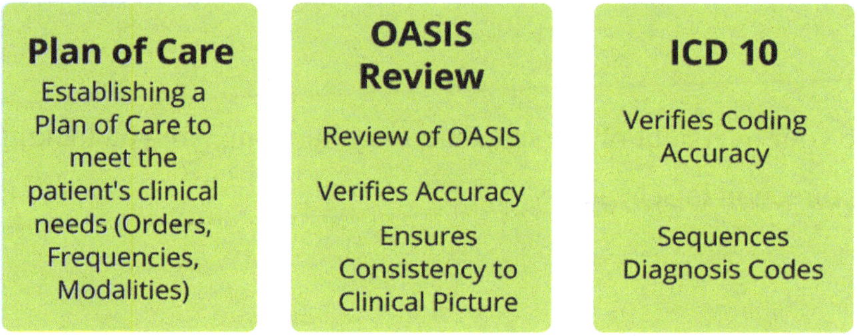

The care team is where much happens all day, every day. This is your bread and butter as a clinical manager. This is your home plate. Establishing processes for consistent oversight and moving the workflows forward.

Plan of Care/485

Ideally, the clinical manager is reviewing the plan of care for the new patient (as well as recertification and during case reviews) to ensure that the plan of care is reasonable for the patient's presentation and clinical need.

- Do you have routine meetings with the team & individually? This is very helpful and a best practice to help enable review of alignment with regulation, appropriate and effective use of resources to achieve good outcomes. Are you performing Case Reviews? Do you review utilization and visit patterns?

- Case reviews are important for the oversight of staffing effectiveness and are vital for inexperienced staff. How are you meeting the needs of inexperienced members of the team? Case reviews offer them such a wealth of information– from learning effective care patterns to ensuring compliance and understanding of the regulations. Is this something you are doing or plan on doing with your teams?

OASIS/Coding

The review of the OASIS/coding to ensure accuracy is vital. This documentation drives both reimbursement and quality measures, which are publicly reported and impact value-based purchasing measures (VBP). It's vital that reimbursement is accurate for the agency.

- What is your current process to ensure the flow of paperwork from clinicians to reviewers? Do you facilitate the workflow?

Ongoing Workflow

- Oversight to the schedule is huge as it drives all the activity for the agency. How are you doing this? Do you think it's effective? Does it give you insight? Do you have ways in which you can engage the team in self-scheduling and controlling the plan of care for their patients? Are you assuring continuity with the staff visiting the patients?

- Are you reviewing documentation for content, supporting eligibility and clinical approach? If not, how can you accommodate for this?

- How are you ensuring that the documentation is efficient and the workdays for the team are efficient and timely? Are they using the technology to its best use, or are they documenting after hours at home? If so, what can you do to fix this?

Business Processes

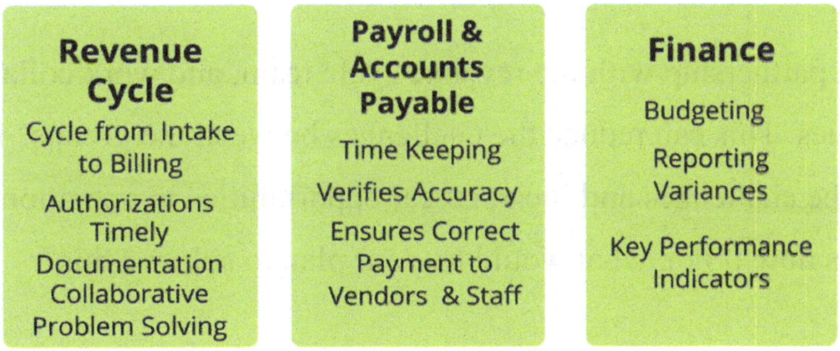

Revenue Cycle

The clinical manager has oversight for many of the steps in the revenue cycle and can influence how well the process is functioning for the organization.

- How are you getting involved in the revenue cycle processes to help resolve issues with missing or late documentation, or visits without authorization? What is your plan to get engaged?

- Establish partnership with the revenue cycle team, and work collaboratively to solve issues. This can reduce the challenges between the groups. This enables you to learn the challenges and it can reveal opportunities in operations. How are you doing this now if not, what would be your plan to achieve this?

Payroll and Accounts Payable

These processes are time bound and require timely attention from the clinical manager to efficiently process.

- Plan for the routine schedule of payroll and accounts payable. Make your time available during the time crunches to get the payroll processes completed in your organization. Block off your calendar, and if out of the office, make sure you are establishing coverage for these processes. Review your planning to get these processes done timely.

Finance

The clinical manager is engaged in several aspects of the finance processes. Budgeting and financial reports are two areas where the clinical manager needs to have involvement.

- Take part in the budget processes, and if able, take time with the finance team to understand how they project the budget. Establish a routine to review the financial reports when they are published to review any variances. Dig into the details with your manager and/or finance manager to understand the causes of any variances and develop a strategy to address if needed. Describe your plans to implement these best practices.

Quality & Compliance Processes

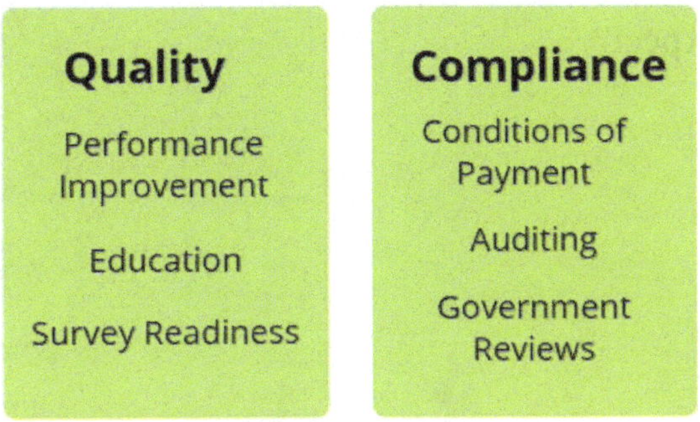

The processes which support quality and compliance will often involve the clinical manager. Most of the processes involve the review of clinical record documentation to assess a variance in quality outcomes, or to assess compliance with regulation and the conditions of payment. In many organizations, different departments and different individuals have oversight in these areas. However, when they converge at the clinical manager level, the activities for each area are very similar and can overlap, as the clinical manager has responsibility and oversight for the quality of care and compliance with regulation.

- Review your organization's QAPI plan. What are the areas that the organization is focusing on? Does your role play a part in that? How can you take part and influence better outcomes?

- What is your role in the survey preparation process? Do you know what to expect on survey? Have you reviewed the interpretive guidance of surveyors to get an idea of what to expect?

- Build a relationship with your quality and compliance teams. Get to know who they are, and how you can use them as a resource. Important to align with goals and activities. Do you know who is handling your agency's quality? Do you know who is overseeing your agency's compliance?

- Remember that compliance is not an event–it should be in the day to day routine. Teaching, overseeing and guidance on regulation and eligibility. What can you do on a day-to-day basis to ensure that your team is always in compliance?

Putting It All Together

Organization

Daily Tasks

Identify for yourself what tasks require your attention every day. These can include;

- Oversight to the team schedule for the day and the week.
- Reading and responding to emails.
- Responding to daily tasks/reviews in the clinical documentation software.
- Reviewing any daily reports–missed visits, documentation, etc.

- How are you organizing your day? Describe or list how you plan to go about your day. If you are currently doing this, describe what you would like to do better and what your challenges are?

Weekly & Monthly Tasks

- Use your calendar to plan ahead
    - Block out time on your calendar for critical tasks
    - Schedule caseload reviews–home supervisions, performance evaluations
- Payroll processes
    - Plan the time it takes to complete

- Describe how you are planning ahead for the things you know must happen in the week and month. Are you planning for payroll? Are you planning and scheduling caseload reviews? What other things should you block out time for.

Meetings

Meetings should be a time where a group of people get together to discuss specific agenda items and to communicate or make decisions. As a clinical manager, you are going to have meetings with your team and meetings with your superiors. For both types of meetings, it is beneficial to be prepared and be on time both for the meeting and when conducting the meeting. Building an agenda with items that need to be addressed during the meeting will assist you to stay on track and to help move others along in the conversation.

- How would you rate yourself for managing meetings? Is there room for improvement in how you manage, plan and conduct the meetings? What is the plan to improve this?

KPIS

Develop a process to review your team's performance for yourself that coincides with the production of the key Performance Indicators (KPI) reports from finance. Schedule in when you expect to receive them and take the time to review and understand your team's performance. This can include setting up standing meetings with a leader from the finance department and/or your supervisor to ensure you are reviewing and responding to the data appropriately. Taking this approach will enable quick attention to anything out of sync with benchmarks, budgets or goals and establish you as a proactive manager in the eyes of leadership.

- How are you reviewing the KPIs for your team? Do you have a set time, and process to ensure you understand what they mean and the action to take to correct any negative variances?

Professionalism

One thing that can really kill your career is being unprofessional. You may be the best manager performing at the highest standard, but if you are unprofessional or a jerk, you will not advance in your career and people will not want to deal with you. Upper leadership would rather deal with someone who was a charm to be around and would take a lesser performing individual if that was the choice.

- Ask yourself honestly how are you doing on the professionalism spectrum, how do you think others are viewing you? How is your self-presentation? How is your work presented? How well organized are you, can others count on you to have done the work? How is your overall demeanor, do you respect others and are you respected? How is your emotional intelligence and self-control?

Taking Care of Yourself

Re-Charging

As a clinical manager, in a sometimes very stressful job, you need to identify when it's time to take care of yourself. We're not superhuman people, and we need to make sure that we acknowledge that. Time away from work is necessary. We need rest, nutrition and peace. Periodically stepping away from the stress of the job is necessary to maintain balance. As clinicians, we think of ourselves as superhuman, that we can take care of everybody and everything and ignore our own needs. It doesn't work that way. We're don't have an endless supply of energy and attention.

- What is your re-charge plan? As a clinician, you really do know what to do here, but I'll ask anyway😊. How do you plan to balance your work life and personal life? Do you take time away and plan to take vacations and time off? Do you take time to step away from work during the week, to give yourself time to re-charge? Describe how you are doing this and what you will do to make it work better for you if need be.

- Re-charging can also mean re-charging your enthusiasm for work by getting professional inspiration. What is your plan to re-charge professionally?

Healthy Living

We know that eating healthy food, getting exercise and enough rest makes us feel great and capable of taking on the world. But we rarely do this well and it takes constant attention. This I know personally, as I have started exercises programs and diet programs hundreds of times, I keep trying though as I still strive to be healthy.

- How are you ensuring you eat right, get enough exercise and rest? If not, how would you plan to ensure you are taking care of your physical self?

Alcohol & Drugs

Be honest with yourself about how you depend on other substances to manage stress. This doesn't work well by the way, it usually complicates things.

- Ask yourself if this is something that needs your attention. What is your plan to address?

Creating Your Career Workplan

The goal of all of this was to learn but also develop a personal plan for your own career growth, whether you're a new manager or your plan is to stay and grow in your current position, or if it's being the CEO of your own agency. Identifying where you need to grow and learn is the first step, and then creating a plan for how to address the areas that need attention would be next. I want to point out that no one who is an outstanding leader has ever felt they have arrived. They continue to focus on areas of professional and personal development. You should try to emulate that behavior, grow and learn, it will help you better enjoy the work and to help others.

Set Your Goals

- Set your goal down in writing. Where do you want to go? How do you want to be? Where do you want to work? How much do you want to make? Refer to the beginning where we discussed your long-term and short-term goals, have they changed?

What is the Plan to Get There?

- What do you need to get there? What skills do you need? What knowledge do you need to have? Do you need to have a further degree? How are you going to do these things, be clear with yourself and specific, such as planning to take a course, or go to a conference that is offering what you are looking for, etc.

What is the Timeline?

- Outline for yourself not only what you will do to achieve your goals but also the plan and timeline for getting there. By when will you take a course? By when will you get a degree?

Re-visit and Re-adjust

Planning doesn't end here. Set a time on your calendar to review your career workplan. This is your ever evolving career plan, treating your career as you would a business will help you drive it forward. We are ever evolving human beings, don't be surprised as things change. Re-adjust the plan, but keep it moving forward!

- Have you set a time to review your plan? What steps will you take to make sure you are looking at this at least every 6 months?

Resources for Growth

There are not a lot of specific resources for the home health or hospice clinical manager for career growth. There can be generic or hospital-based resources in books and courses. It was this unavailability of resources that prompted the creation of these courses and The Clinical Manager Source. Review your state and national home health and hospice organizations for additional training and conferences.

At *The Clinical Manager Source* www.theclinicalmanagersource.com we offer resources to fill in the missing links for home health and hospice managers. Our podcasts offer general and specific insight into what the clinical manager needs to know. The Premium Podcast, *The Clinical Manager Source* is by subscription only–but is very cheap–to hear commercial free segments on operations best practices and guests who are industry experts offering their own professional insight into the clinical manager world and career insight from their specific experiences. It's like having a coffee with your own consultant, and about as expensive as the coffee would cost!

We offer a more general industry insight podcast *Coffee & Conversation*, with commercials from sponsors, that discuss current issues impacting the industry. If you subscribe to the Premium Podcast, you will have this available without the commercials, and prior to the public release!

As part of this course, you have access to be admitted into the Private Facebook group, for *The Clinical Manager Source* https://www.facebook.com/groups/406944398174840 where you will have access to other colleagues across the country, as well as the administrator for the group (me and other industry experts).

Appendix

Deep Dive Regulations - Answers

Name the 5 requirements for certification of a patient in home health, what are the requirements?

1. Home Bound
2. Skilled/Medically Necessary
3. Under the care of a physician or allowed provider
4. Has a plan of care established and periodically reviewed by a physician or allowed provider
5. Had a face to face in the allowed time frames for reasons they are on home health

The Criteria for Home Bound

- For a patient to be eligible to receive covered home health services under both Part A and Part B, the law requires that a physician or allowed practitioner certify in all cases that the patient is confined to his/her home.
- For purposes of the statute, an individual shall be considered "confined to the home" (homebound) if the following two criteria are met:
  - 1. Criterion One: The patient must either: - Because of illness or injury, need the aid of supportive devices such as crutches, canes, wheelchairs, and walkers; the use of special transportation; or the assistance of another person in order to leave their place of residence **OR**

- Have a condition such that leaving his or her home is medically contraindicated. If the patient meets one of the criterion one conditions, then the patient must ALSO meet two additional requirements defined in criterion two below.
    - 2. Criterion Two: - There must exist a normal inability to leave home; AND - Leaving home must require a considerable and taxing effort.

Source: Medicare Benefit Policy Manual, Chapter 7, Home Health Services at: https://www.cms.gov/files/document/se19027.pdf

What are some things that a skilled nurse can do under home health? (Chapter 7 - Section 40.1) (Specific examples are in the Medicare Benefit Policy Manual– Chapter 7)

- Observation and assessment
- Teaching and training
- Treatment
- Medication administration (requiring the skills of a nurse)
- Management and evaluation of the Plan of Care
    - *Underlying conditions or complications require that only a registered nurse can ensure that essential unskilled care is achieving its purpose.*
        - Source: Medicare Benefit Policy Manual, Chapter 7, Home Health Services at: https://www.cms.gov/files/document/se19027.pdf

What is it about a patient's condition that would qualify them for skilled therapy services rather than just having a home health aide do exercises with a patient? (Chapter 7 40.2.1)

"*The service of a physical therapist, speech-language pathologist, or occupational therapist is a skilled therapy service if the inherent complexity of the service is such that it can be performed safely and/or effectively only by or under the general supervision of a skilled therapist. To be covered, assuming all other eligibility and coverage criteria have been met, the skilled services must also be reasonable and necessary to the treatment of the patient's illness or injury or to the restoration or maintenance of function affected by the patient's illness or injury. It is necessary to determine whether individual therapy services are skilled and whether, in view of the patient's overall condition, skilled management of the services provided is needed."* **40.2.1 includes further reading to further lay out the requirements for therapy services in home health**. *Be sure to read these.*

Source: Medicare Benefit Policy Manual, Chapter 7, Home Health Services at: https://www.cms.gov/files/document/se19027.pdf

Orders–The order is missing duration of care. *SN 2 to 3 x a week* ***for 4 weeks*** *for assessment of cardiac status, lung sounds, vitals and medication teaching of new prescriptions.*

References

Belker, Loren B., McCormick, Jim., Topchik, Gary. *The First-Time Manager, 7th Edition*. Harper Collins Leadership, 2018

HHA Center Webpage at: http://www.cms.gov/Center/Provider-Type/Home-Health-Agency-HHA-Center.html

Marrelli, Tina. *The Nurse Manager's Survival Guide, 4th Edition*. Indianapolis: Sigma Theta Tau International, 2018

Medicare Benefit Policy Manual, Chapter 7, Home Health Services at: https://www.cms.gov/files/document/se19027.pdf

MLN Matters Number: SE19027. (2019). *Overview of the Patient Driven Groupings Model.* Department of Health & Human Services.

PDGM Webpage at: https://www.cms.gov/Medicare/Medicare-Fee-for-Service-Payment/HomeHealthPPS/HH-PDGM

Potter, James. Kavanagh, Mike. *The Successful Manager*. Potter Consulting LLC, 2020

The HRmeister. (2017, October 29). *Essential Elements of Employee Retention.* Retrieved from Lynchburg Regional SHRM: https://lrshrm.shrm.org/blog/2017/10/essential-elements-employee-retention

Made in the USA
Monee, IL
02 November 2026

67383311R00050